30-DAY
SOCIAL MEDIA
DETOX

☐ No Facebook until 12pm.

HOW DO YOU FEEL?

- [ ] Delete all unused apps.

HOW DO YOU FEEL?

- [ ] No social media updates today!

HOW DO YOU FEEL?

☐ No phone during meal times.

HOW DO YOU FEEL?

DAY 5

- [ ] No social media scrolling till 11am.

HOW DO YOU FEEL?

DAY 6

☐ Call a friend today— don't just stalk.

HOW DO YOU FEEL?

DAY 7

- [ ] Twitter free day!

HOW DO YOU FEEL?

DAY 8

Meditate 15-20min Phone free.

HOW DO YOU FEEL?

DAY 9

- [ ] Put your phone in a seperate room at bedtime.

HOW DO YOU FEEL?

DAY 10

Spend 2h phone free with someone.

HOW DO YOU FEEL?

DAY 11

☐ No Facebook all day!

HOW DO YOU FEEL?

DAY 12

- [ ] Limit of 20min social media today.

HOW DO YOU FEEL?

HOW DO YOU FEEL?

DAY 13

- [ ] No status updates today!

HOW DO YOU FEEL?

☐ Walk for 1h outside.

HOW DO YOU FEEL?

HOW DO YOU FEEL?

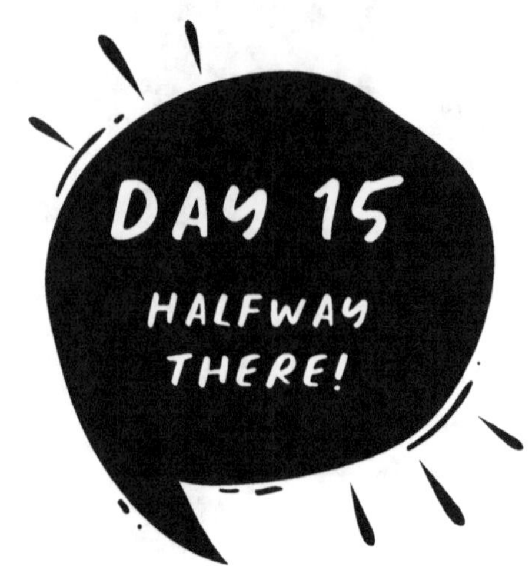

No social media all day!

HOW DO YOU FEEL?

DAY 16

No phone
at meals
all day!

HOW DO YOU FEEL?

HOW DO YOU FEEL?

DAY 17

- [ ] Laptop & phone off by 6pm.

HOW DO YOU FEEL?

DAY 18

- [ ] **30min social media limit.**

HOW DO YOU FEEL?

HOW DO YOU FEEL?

- Exercise phone free today.

HOW DO YOU FEEL?

DAY 20

☐ No
Insta
all day!

HOW DO YOU FEEL?

- 20min social media limit.

HOW DO YOU FEEL?

DAY 22

☐ Read a book for 45min.

HOW DO YOU FEEL?

DAY 23

- [ ] No social media scrolling till 3pm.

HOW DO YOU FEEL?

HOW DO YOU FEEL?

DAY 24

☐ No social media after 5pm.

HOW DO YOU FEEL?

DAY 25

- [ ] **15min social media limit.**

HOW DO YOU FEEL?

DAY 26

- [ ] Zero social media today.

HOW DO YOU FEEL?

- [ ] Suprise a loved one. No phone today.

HOW DO YOU FEEL?

- [ ] No phone after work/ school.

HOW DO YOU FEEL?

DAY 29

- [ ] Set up future goals. No phone for 1h.

HOW DO YOU FEEL?

DAY 30

☐ Your choice— challenge yourself!

HOW DO YOU FEEL?

HOW DO YOU FEEL?

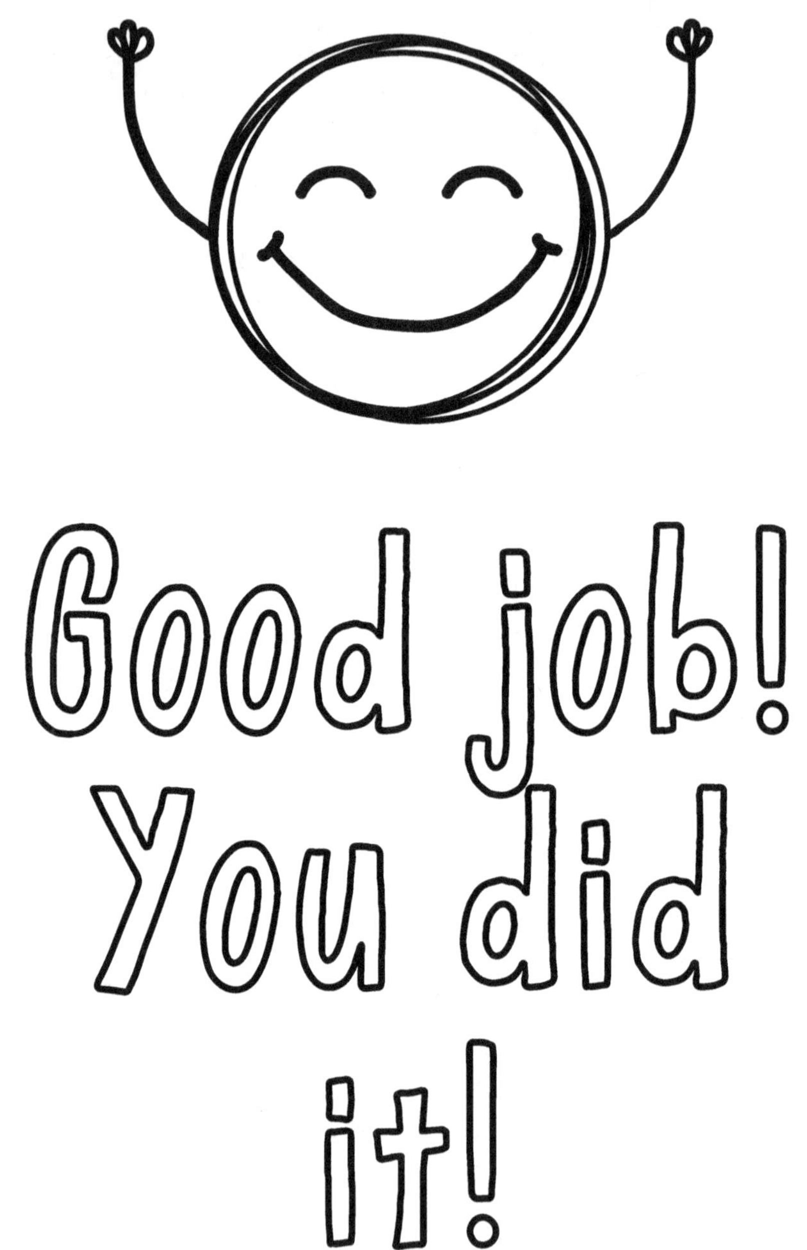
Good job! You did it!

HOW DO YOU FEEL?

HOW DO YOU FEEL?

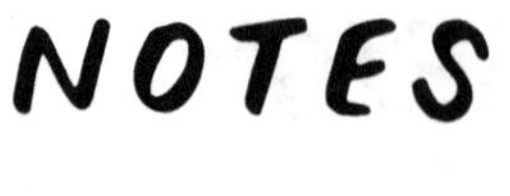

NOTES

NOTES

NOTES

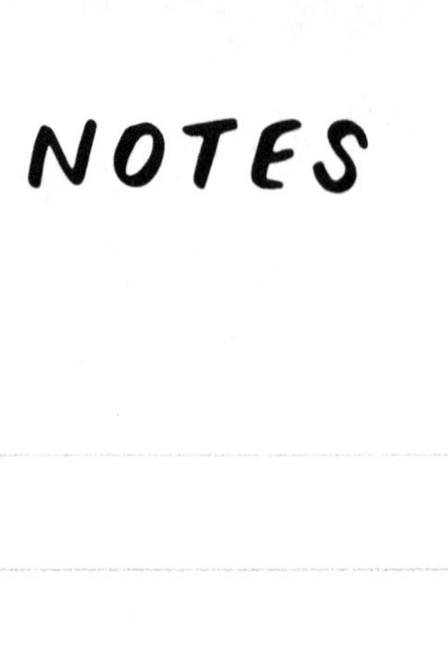

NOTES

NOTES

NOTES

NOTES

NOTES

NOTES

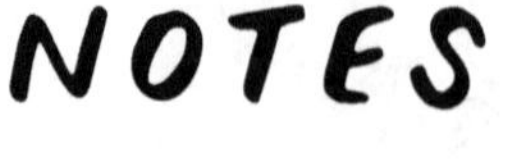

NOTES

NOTES

NOTES

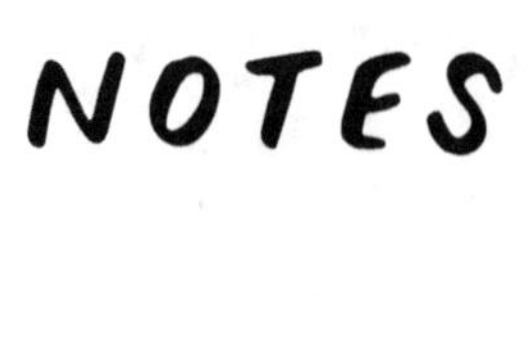
NOTES

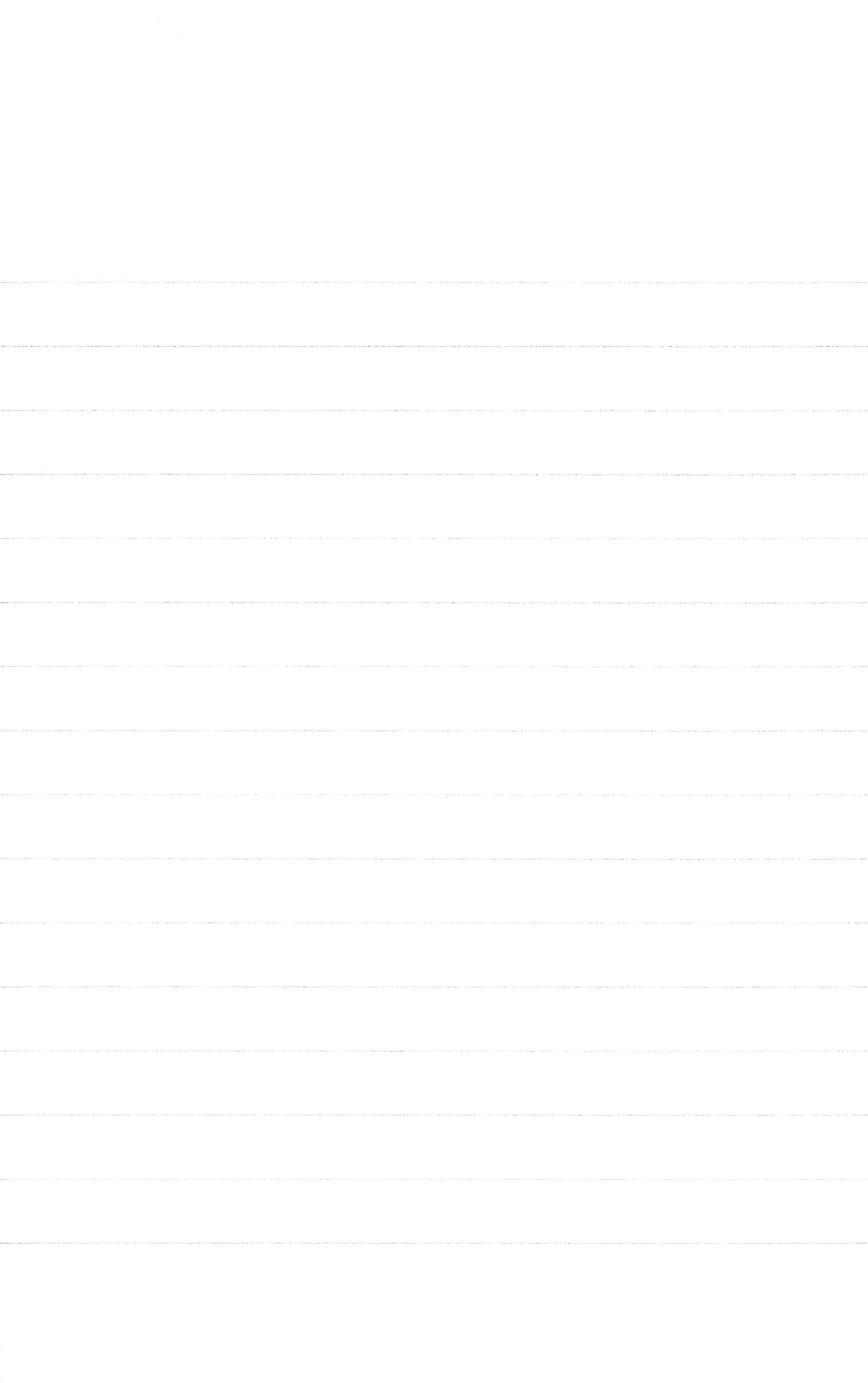

NOTES

NOTES

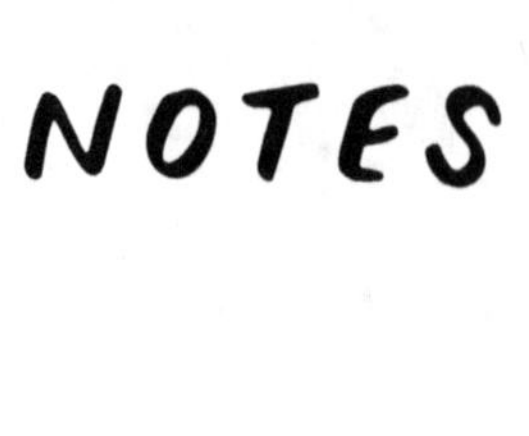

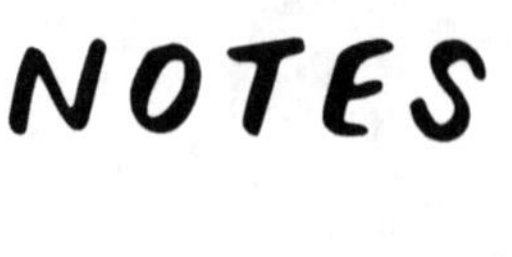

NOTES

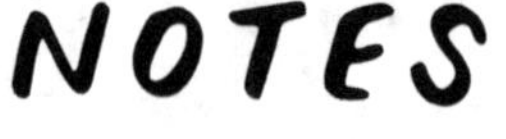